What Is Good Hair?

Thembekile Dube

ISBN 979-8-88751-621-9 (paperback)
ISBN 979-8-88751-623-3 (hardcover)
ISBN 979-8-88751-622-6 (digital)

Christian Faith Publishing
832 Park Avenue
Meadville, PA 16335
www.christianfaithpublishing.com

Printed in the United States of America

This book is dedicated to myself, Thembekile Dube, for all of the times you gazed in the mirror and questioned your beauty because of the condition of the plant on your head.

I also dedicate this to any and every one who needs more love. You got this!

Special dedication to my beautiful mother, Sithabile Mathwasa. I wouldn't be here without you.

Introduction

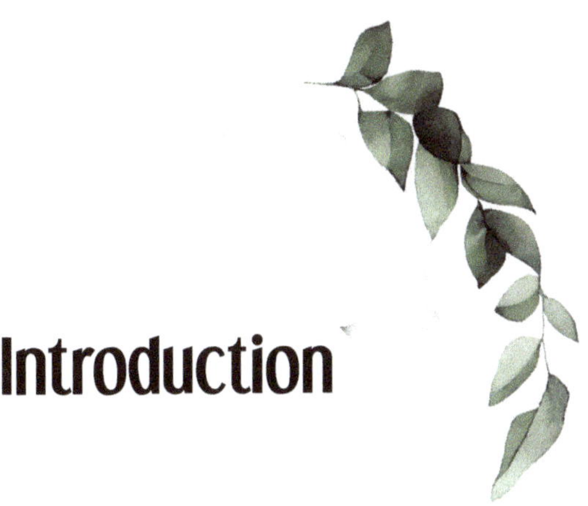

Growing up in a black home, regardless of gender, hair is bound to be a subject of importance in one's daily life. The idea of leaving the house "not looking crazy" is drilled into our minds by those who want the best for us. This idea of "looking crazy" often centers around our clothes and hair alike. Unlike clothing, hair can only be altered so much in order to fit the beauty standards, or at minimum to not look crazy. So alter we often do, until the locks on our heads share some resemblance to those of individuals blessed to be born with "good hair."

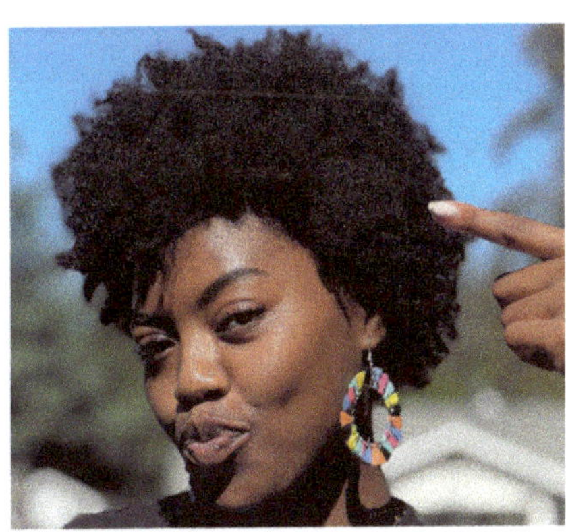

As a child with naturally very thick 4C hair, I quickly came to terms with the fact that waking up and walking out of the house with my hair in near natural state (water and comb) would be the very equivalent of what many black mothers would describe as looking crazy. I expeditiously discovered the magnificence that is the "creamy crack" inside a pretty and pink "just for me" box at the tender age of five. I watched as my hair transitioned from free, bountiful curls to elongated, thinner, and more manageable strands as the chemical concoction penetrated my locks and eventually made it to my scalp where my indication that it had done its job was a burning sensation that wouldn't be terminated until it was finally washed out of my hair. Then *bam*! Just like that, I was transformed from "lookin crazy" to being pretty and presentable. And albeit my hair still didn't fit the criteria for "good hair," I was made aware that it was significantly better than the state in which it began.

Perms were just one of the many ways I would discover that could elevate the beauty of my hair. In middle school, when my father learned of the contents within those pretty pink magic boxes, he informed my sister and I that it was no longer an option for us (well as long as it was coming out of his pocket). My world was rocked in a way that brought into question so many things about myself. How was I to maintain beauty when the one thing helping me attain that was taken away from me? I dreaded having to become natural so much so that I preferred watching my hair shed and going through those awkward phases of transition than to just cut off the damage.

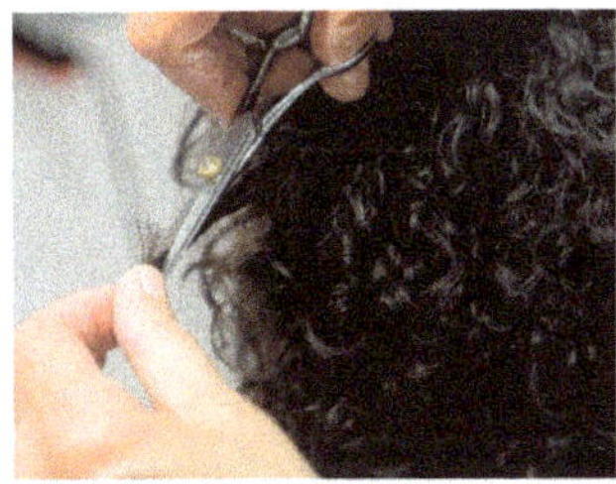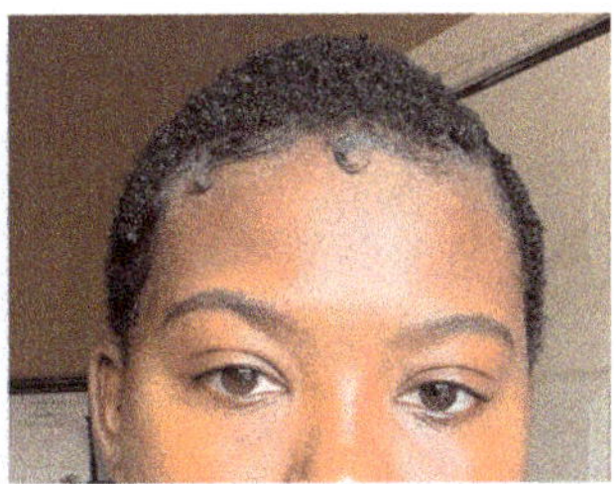

The trepidation that came over my entire being when the thought of becoming natural crossed my mind occurred not only because of my opinion on natural hair (especially the kind I had on my head) not being beautiful but also because I had absolutely no idea how to take care of it. I didn't even know many adult women in my life who actually had natural hair to use as a template. At that time, braids became my best friend. Now that I was older and my dad was finally okay with me getting box braids instead of just cornrows without added hair. I was really unstoppable once I learned how to do them to myself!

By the time I got to college, I had been natural for approximately six years. I had much more knowledge and understanding of natural hair than when I was forced into my natural hair journey all those years ago. That knowledge had helped me start seeing the beauty of natural hair and feel comfortable spending time with mine. When I wanted to go out looking *GOODT*, my wig was the first thing I made sure to plop on. I was still going to need some time before I could look at the kind of hair coming from my scalp and see it as "presentable" in all settings, especially ones that involve me looking my best or classy (if you will).

My hair journey, similarly to many black children, did not start on my own. With influences from parents, aunties, stepmothers, family friends, friends, and beauticians, I was taught many different standards of beauty and what was needed in order for me to fit that mold. From perms to blowouts, silk presses, braids, and wigs, I was fully equipped with an arsenal of weapons I could use in the never-ending war I was waging with my natural hair. And wage war I did—until I finally got tired of fighting.

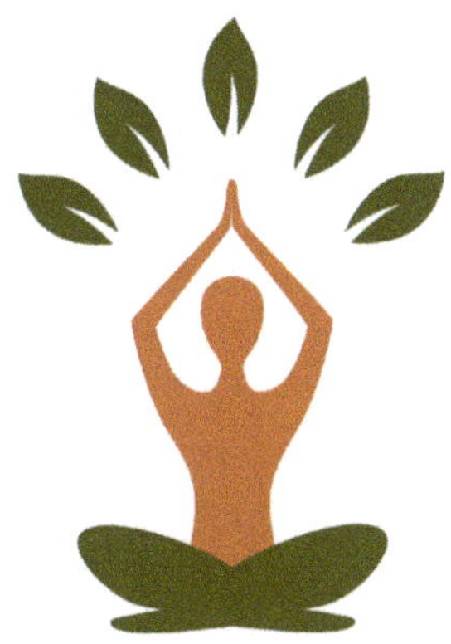

The End of the Battle

In 2020, ten years after I first became natural, I finally put my weapons down. I came to realize that there is no need for me to fight what/who I am naturally and that even if I did, I wasn't going to win. As my dad always says, "Knowledge is power," so seek knowledge I have done. Lots of YouTube videos and articles later, I became equipped with a new set of tools: oils, techniques, moisturizers, routines, styles, and most importantly confidence. These would be the tools I used and continue to use to fortify my relationship with my hair and alter my misconstrued ideas of beauty.

After over two years of extensive research and a whole lot of trial and error, I am ready to share the knowledge I have accrued with those who might be able to relate to my story in any way or even those who are just interested in natural hair and hair care.

In the pages to come, I will share with you the true meaning of "good hair." You will learn not only how to take care of natural hair but also how to grow it as well as how to repair it. Together we will also dismantle the many myths about natural hair care (i.e., we don't need water in our hair). For those scientists like myself, I also include the scientific facts that correlate to the subject matter at hand.

Above all else, I pray that my words will fill you with a sense of peace when you think of taking care of your natural hair and an overwhelming sense of love when you look at yourself in the mirror independently from whatever state your hair is in (relaxed, natural, curly, straight, done, or on the top of your head). True beauty resides within your being and cannot be quantified by anyone outside of yourself.

Where the Term Comes From

Let's begin with dismantling what "good hair" isn't.

Good hair is not the quality of hair deemed to be "acceptable" in the eyes of a society blinded by the white standards, which have been implemented into all cultures during the cross contamination, which occurred during slavery, colonization, and precolonization. Black people have experienced a tormentful history at the hands of white people; the physical scars run deeper than the flesh, but mental wounds exemplify the epitome of torture we endured at their merciless, blood-stained hands. Those lacerations have completely altered the true nature of black minds so much that our standards of what is "good," "beautiful," and "acceptable" have shifted to things, traits, and beings outside of those found within black people and our culture.

Together as a community, we must redefine what is "good" and "beautiful" for the sake of our mental well-being and that of our children and their children for generations to come. My goal is to assist you in this journey by introducing you to what "good hair" truly is.

Redefining and Identifying What Our Standards Are

Our concept of normalcy and/or the standards of what is "good/acceptable" begins formulating in our minds during youth. The visuals we see, the messages we hear, and the lessons we are taught validate the legitimacy of these standards. As we age, we continue to receive affirmation of these standards we were long ago taught; at some point, these standards have transformed into beliefs. Beliefs are firmly held opinions, in other words, thoughts that we keep thinking.

In order to redefine our standards of beauty, we must first shift our beliefs, or we must start thinking new thoughts. These thoughts should hold yourself as the standard of your beauty.

The start of your day is very crucial in determining the tone/mood of the rest of the day, so it is important to take time at the onset of the day to set your intentions. Setting your intentions could be visualization or something as simple as "I am" statements. These statements aid in the reprogramming of our mind and of our misconstrued belief system.

Take a moment to settle your breathing. Stand facing a mirror (optional). Say the first statement. Take a deep breath. Release. Say the next statement. Continue.

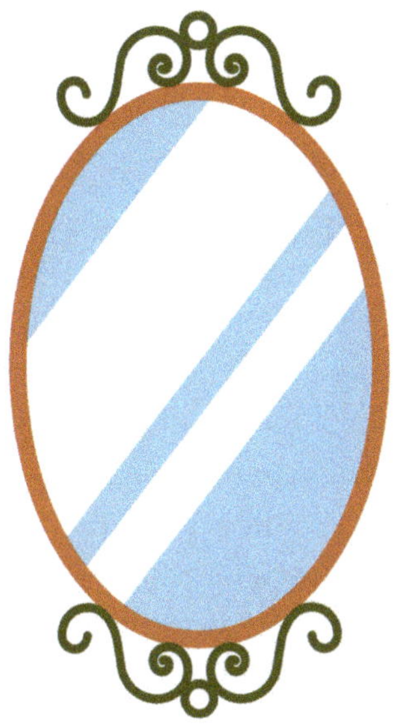

Affirming My Beauty

~ I am beautiful.
~ I am loving and deserving of love.
~ I am the standard of my beauty.
~ I love my morning face.
~ I have a beautiful smile.
~ I am grateful for all of my attractive features.
~ I have gorgeous eyes that reflect my pure soul.
~ People find me extremely attractive.

Affirming My Hair

~ I love my hair.
~ I only compare my hair to the way it was yesterday.
~ I appreciate my hair the way it is.
~ I enjoy learning my hair.
~ I am at my goal length.
~ I am grateful for the individuality of each strand.
~ I take great care of my hair.
~ I love my hair in every state.
~ My hair is luscious and soft to the touch.
~ I love my strong, healthy, and shiny hair.
~ It feels natural and easy to grow my hair.
~ My hair only adds to the beauty I already possess inside and out.
~ My hair is naturally thick, strong, and beautiful.
~ I eat a healthy and balanced diet to keep my hair healthy and nourished.
~ My expectations of hair growth are realistic and individual to myself.

Take these statements as they resonate to you. If you feel resistance while reading one, skip over it, and come back when it feels more natural or "believable" to you. Create a regimen that feels good to you and includes time spent loving you.

Pro tip: Don't stop when you start feeling good! Consistency is a must here.

Chapter 1

What Is Good Hair?

Good hair is the hair that comes out of your scalp.

Take a look in the mirror. No, really, *stand up, and look in the mirror.*

Do you see your hair? I don't care what state it is currently in. Take a moment, and truly appreciate the hair on your head.

Now that you have seen your hair, you now know what good hair is. You didn't need me to tell you what good hair is because it is, and always will be, the hair that is on your head.

I think most of us now have a name for our hair; if you don't, maybe now is a good time to name him or her; with a personality of her own, I had to name mine as well. Her name is "Plant," and she has taught me so much (a lot of which I'll be sharing with you in the pages to come). Plant received her name two years ago, when I finally had a solid understanding of how to take care of her. During the process of getting to know her, I learned her likes, dislikes, what makes her grow, and what breaks her down. The whole journey taught me that hair is comparable to a plant, in the way it should be cared for and maintained as well as its individuality.

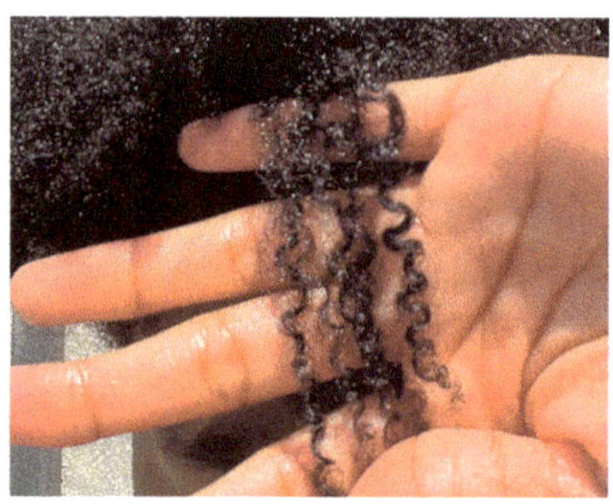

There is no one kind of leaf that sets the standard for what beauty is within the category of flora. In fact, it is the vast variety of the leaves that often enhance the overall beauty and allure of a plant. Similarly, your hair is just as idiosyncratic; it is beautiful because it is unique to you and only you.

Chapter 2

Clean Hair

How clean should the hair be? Your hair does not need to be sparkling clean every day; in fact, it shouldn't be. It is normal to have small amounts of dandruff in your hair because dandruff is dead skin cells. Just like all other cells in your body, the skin on your head also dies after a period of time. Unlike the cells on most other parts of your body, even bodily skin, the skin cells on our head, are a lot more noticeable when they die, especially on darker-colored hair, because of their white color. But don't be alarmed. This is a natural process and should not harm you; if anything, it might cause a little embarrassment, but you can shake that off just like the dandruff.

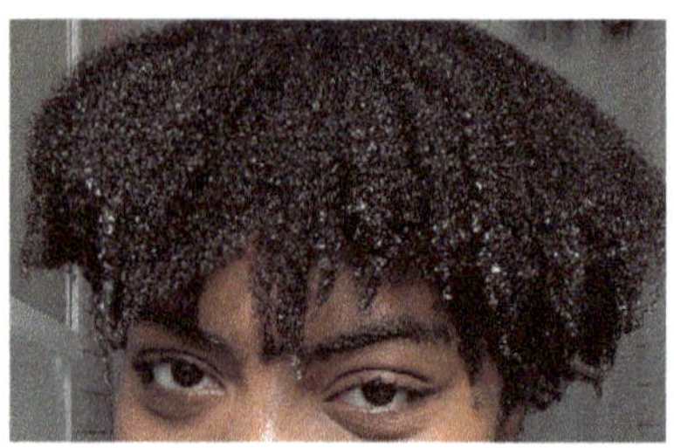

The following are tips for managing dandruff:

1. Get to know your scalp. What does it need? In what conditions does it flourish the most?
    a. For myself, I know that my scalp flourishes the most in well-oiled conditions. My scalp loves to be fed, so I make sure to keep it full with a balance of oils and greases.

2. Know when it is time to cleanse your scalp.
    a. When it comes to the accumulation of dead skin and buildup, it is important to know how much is too much. You know your hair better than anyone else, so with time and practice, you'll be able to spot just when is the right time to cleanse the hair and scalp.
    b. It is important not to allow too much buildup to accumulate on the scalp because that prevents the nutrients in the oils from penetrating the scalp. It also is like clogged pores. We know clogged pores on the face lead to breakouts and generally less clear

skin, so be considerate of the pores on your scalp. They need to be open in order to breathe and properly function as well.

    c.   Don't overdo it. Washing your hair too much can lead to overly dry and brittle hair. Shampoo rids the hair of oils, a lot of which are naturally occurring and good for the hair and scalp, so maintaining a balance of just enough oil is essential for hair maintenance and health.

    d.   I personally wash my hair once every week and a half or every two and a half weeks, depending on the style.

3.   Get to know about dandruff maintenance products.

    a.   There are a variety of dandruff maintenance and dandruff-reducing products on the market today, from shampoos to creams and moisturizer to DIY products you can make at home.

    b.   Henna—a product I speak highly of with its many benefits for natural hair. One use for henna is dandruff management with its excellent antifungal properties.

Chapter 3

Strong Hair

Because hair is made of proteins, it is pertinent that we maintain the health of those proteins in order to keep the bonds strong and together in order to prevent breakage.

There are a plethora of treatments already made and available for purchase online and in store. I prefer the natural treatments made from ingredients available in a home kitchen. Below you will find one of my favorite protein-enriching hair treatments.

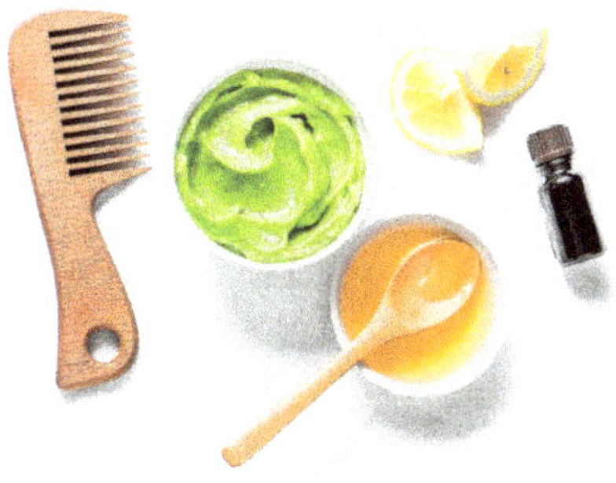

Here is my favorite at-home protein treatment:

Ingredients: egg, mayo, avocado oil, and banana (Add an avocado for even more protein.)

The amount depends on the length and thickness of hair. The following are the ingredients for medium-length hair:

- 1 Egg—eggs contain vitamins A and E, biotin, and folate, which lead to thick and healthy hair. The fats in the yolk promote hair growth and therefore are great for length, with a bonus of added shine.

- ⅓ Cup Mayo—mayonnaise is filled with proteins, vitamins, and fatty acids, which lead to softer, smoother, and shiner hair because of the intense moisturizing properties of the fatty acids.

- 2 tbsp Avocado Oil—benefits located in chapter 4.

- ¾ Banana—banana contains silica, a mineral element that aids the body in making collagen. Collagen is a protein that leads to stronger and bouncier hair without frizz. Banana also has the added benefit of containing antimicrobial properties which manage dandruff.

Optional: ½ avocado—avocado has a plethora of benefits. It has high fat content, antioxidants, minerals, and anti-inflammatory properties. It is also packed with nutrients such as vitamins C, D, and E, iron, and zinc. Avocado is special in that it is also a "nutrient booster," meaning that it increases the absorption of fat solubles like vitamins A, D, K, and E, which nourish and strengthen the hair, leading to growth. They also aid in hair loss prevention because they unclog the hair follicles.

Instructions: Blend the ingredients together. Wet hair. Apply mask generously from root to tip. Cover with a plastic cap for two hours. Thoroughly rinse and condition.

Strong hair isn't just about maintaining those disulfide bonds with added protein. Another way to maintain those bonds is by simply being gentle with your hair. For us curly hair folks, those curls mean more disulfide bonds, which means more fragility, so the curlier your hair is, the more gentle you need to be with it because it is fragile and can break quite easily.

Being gentle with your hair looks like taking your time when doing and undoing your hair. I know the process of getting a style put in can be lengthy, and we often dread the idea of having to spend an extended amount of time taking it down. This makes it easy to get into the habit of rushing hastily through it to get it out, which often leads to much more breakage than we bargain for. Growth also means length retention, so if growth is the goal, you *MUST* be gentle.

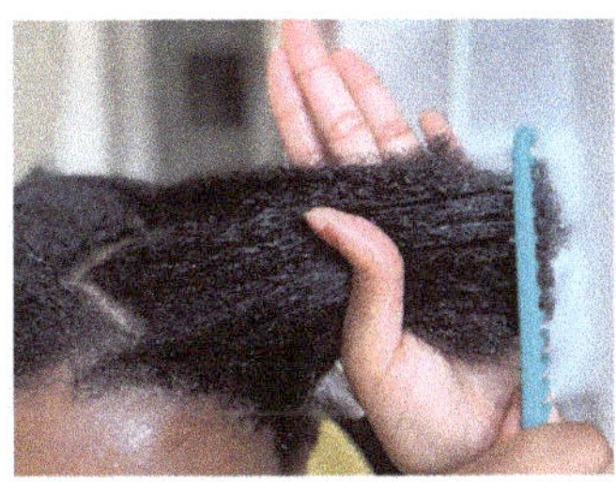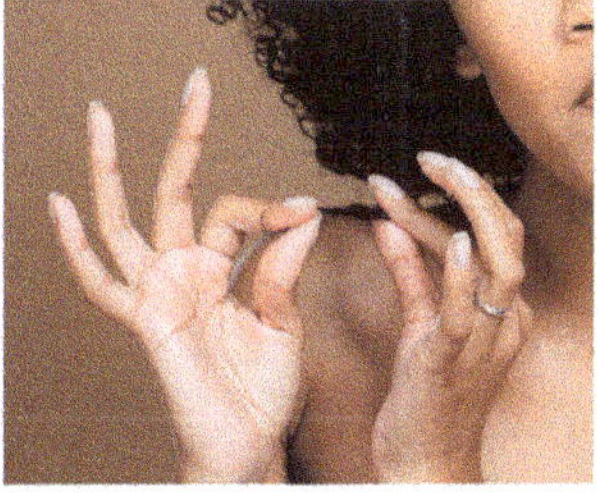

Minimize combing/brushing especially on dry hair. Try donning styles that can be worn for at least five days without combing through the hair. If combing the hair is necessary, wet it to provide the most ease and least amount of friction possible.

Be gentle. Doing natural hair can take time. Your coils can lock onto other coils and create unexpected knots. Take your time working through them, and don't just rip them out.

Chapter 4

Hydrated Hair

A common misconception in the black community is that our hair does not need water (or not very often at least). If we relate back to the analogy of our hair being reminiscent of a plant, we can understand why this cannot be true. The vast majority of plants require a dousing of water on a regular basis—ranging from once a day to once a week. The hair is a plant, the leaves and flowers, and the scalp is the soil where the roots are. Attend to the roots, and water, water, water. Regardless of the style, your hair does need to be watered; the amount or regularity in which you need to water your hair will vary depending on a few factors.

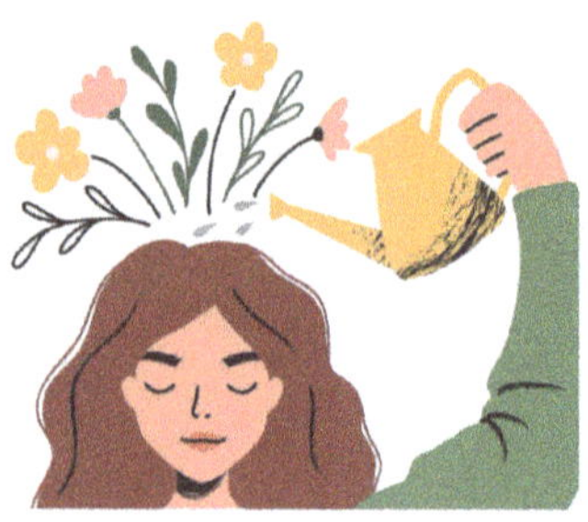

Texture and Porosity

Often, the thicker the hair, the more water is required in order to penetrate the strand and reach the scalp. Low-porosity hair is identical in the fact that more water is required (initially). Low-porosity hair does not allow for water to easily penetrate the hair shaft, so more of it is often required, in addition to techniques that increase water absorption. On the flip side, low-porosity hair holds water very well, so the weekly watering regime might include less watering days than that of someone with high-porosity hair. High porosity differs because albeit it is easy for water to penetrate the hair shaft, it is also just as easy for water to leave. This type of hair might require less water at one time but more frequent watering days.

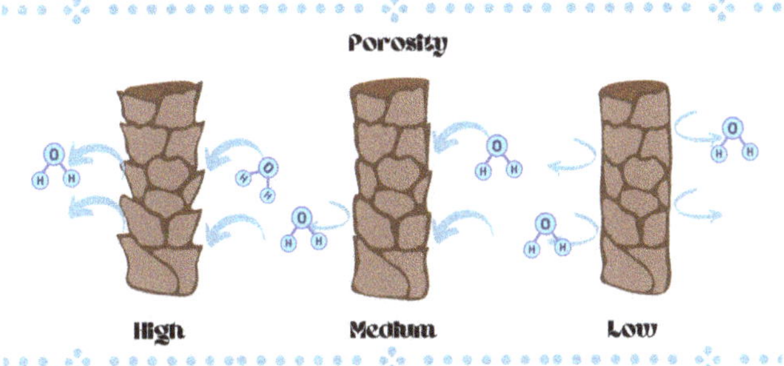

Style

If the hair is in a style exposing more of the scalp, most of the hair is usually "put away" or protected. Styles like this do not require as much water because the hair is usually not drying out as fast (depending on the climate). In contrast, styles in which more of the hair is exposed or "loose" or unprotected, watering more often is essential.

Pro tip: Protective styles, which include weave like box braids, provide even more protection to the hair shaft and therefore require less watering (of the hair shaft) than single braids without weave. But don't forget to water your scalp.

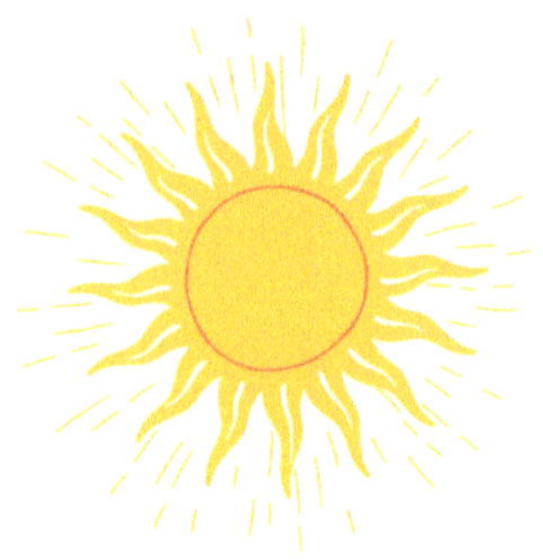

Climate/Weather

Heat has to be divided into two categories because dry heat has different effects on hair than humid heat. Dry heat dries the air, hence reducing the moisture in the air available to replenish the hair. In dry settings, more frequent watering and/or more water is required in order to maintain optimal hair moisture. In humid settings, there is significantly more moisture in the air. So you get your hair watered for *THE FREE*. This climate requires less frequent watering and/or less water in the hair.

Oils/Grease

In addition to H_2O, plants also require fertilizer. Oil and grease act as the fertilizer in the analogy of hair to a plant. In the same way that plants need water, they also need nutrient-rich soil. Greases and oils are applied to the scalp so that they can be absorbed at the root of the hair. Which one to use depends on the hair type and most of all personal preference. I have found that a combination of both works best for my hair. Applying the grease once during the installation of a style and oil throughout the duration of my time with the style keeps my scalp breathable and well nourished.

Hair nourishment and watering go hand in hand for me, even to the extent that when I refer to a "weekly moisturizing regime," I am referring to a routine that includes time for watering and oiling the hair and scalp. Oil behaves as a sealant in its interaction with water. When water is applied to the hair, it is a good idea to follow it up with the application of oil; this will seal the hair shaft, locking the water in and ensuring that it will have time to be absorbed by the cuticle instead of quickly evaporating out.

Not all oils are equally beneficial to the hair and body. Saturated and monounsaturated fats are better able to penetrate the hair than polyunsaturated fats. Some oils fall into the category of essential oils, while others are carrier oils. Carrier oils like olive, almond, jojoba, and coconut oils come from plants and have a neutral smell. Essential oils (such as lavender and rosemary) are distilled from plants and are highly concentrated, leading to more pungent smelling oils. Coating the hair shaft in a thin layer of oil adds to the flexibility of the stand, reducing breakage.

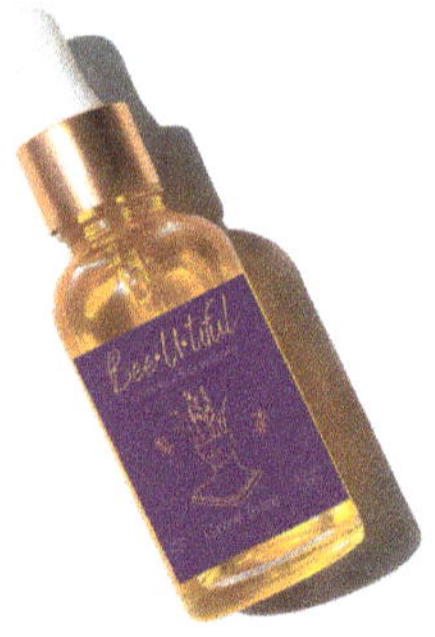

Here are some examples of oils and their benefits:

- Almond—soothes and moisturizes the scalp
- Argan—antioxidants; moisturizes and nourishes
- Avocado—monounsaturated; contains vitamins, minerals, and antioxidants for health and strength
- Coconut—softens hair and increases shine
- Lavender—deeply conditions the hair for added shine and dandruff control
- Rosemary—stimulates roots, increases circulation in the scalp; also for hair growth

In conclusion, it is important to regard your hair as the plant that it is. Treat your hair to water and nourishment often so as to feed it and promote growth. We can all learn how to become plant moms to our most precious plant baby—the one on our heads. Achieving the optimal level of moisture will require trial and error as well as patience (like much of your hair journey). If you find yourself needing inspiration, return to the "Affirming My Hair" section in chapter 2.

Chapter 5

Minimal Breakage

Hair can become damaged from a variety of things—heat, chemicals, pulling/friction, overstyling, or lack of attention. But don't fret. There are plenty of ways to keep those locks safe and in good health! The problems that arise from overstyling and pulling/friction have been discussed in previous chapters, so make sure to reread those sections.

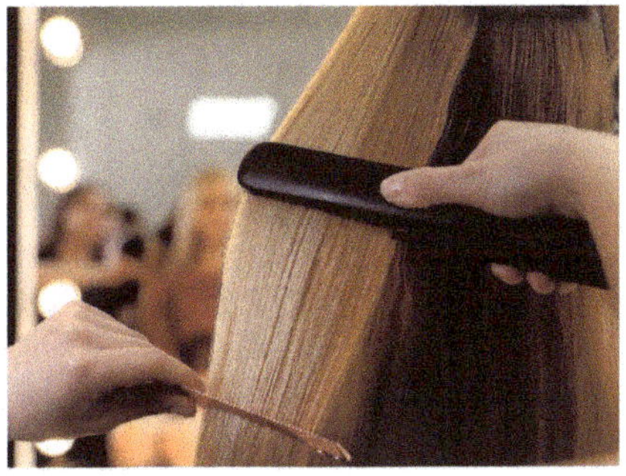

Heat

This brings us back to the scientific explanation of what hair is—proteins. High heat exposure alters the shape of the hair's keratin strands. The alpha keratin is converted to beta keratin, which leads to loss of hair elasticity and hair that is more prone to breakage because of its weaker bonds. This change happens at temperatures over 300°F, which might shock you when considering that most heating tools (i.e., curling irons, flat irons, blow dryers, etc.) have heat settings that reach 400°F.

Heat also affects the topic we just covered in the last chapter—moisture or the lack thereof. The inner part of the hair strand is called the cortex, and it is where the water molecules reside, which are bound to the keratin proteins. The hair's protein structure is changed when heat is applied because the natural oils are stripped from the shaft and the water molecules evaporate. Those excessively high temperatures cause the water to dry rapidly leading to cracked cuticles (the hair's outer layer), making the hair more susceptible to further damage.

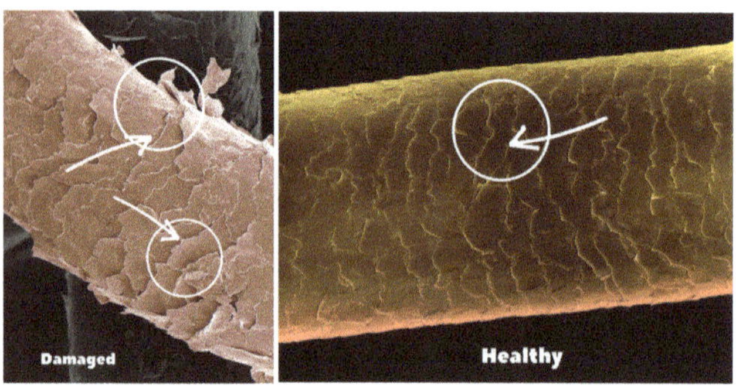

Fix/Repair

Heat damage is a change in the physical structure of the hair by way of chemical bonds, and therefore it is a permanent change. Once heat damage occurs, sadly, there is no repairing it. So what are some possible solutions?

—   Scissors! This involves simply cutting off the damage, not necessarily a big chop, but one that just includes the removal of the damaged strands or sections. This will allow your hair the fresh start it often needs to let health take root. This also frees you from having to tuck in those loose strands that have fallen limp and no longer blend with its more bouncy and lively neighboring strands.

– Maintenance. For those who would prefer to keep their length, maintaining the hair in its current condition is also a possibility. Putting in place measures and routines which allow for moisture retention will keep the hair looking shiny and feeling soft. High-porosity hair can be treated with leave-in conditioners, creams, and oils. It also needs more protein to make up for all that was lost in the damage, so using products with keratin and other proteins is essential.

– Prevention. Preventative measures are a must! They are so much more effective than reactive measures, which attempt to repair what could have been prevented.

Here are some preventive measures I recommend:

1. Avoid using excess heat with hot tools. Aim for a temperature range between 200 and 300°F.

2. Use heat protectant. You can find a variety of heat protectants online and in stores. They can be applied to wet or dry hair and add a layer of protection to your hair prior to the use of heat.

3. Use heating tools wisely. We love a *one past queen*—am I right, ladies! When applying heat to the hair, there is no need to overdo it. A single pass with the heating tool should be sufficient enough to achieve the style you desire. There is absolutely no need to flat iron the same piece of hair three times before moving onto the next piece. If you find yourself having to do this, it might be time to consider the quality of tools you are purchasing. A quote from my Aunt Queen says, "Cheap is expensive." It is important to weigh the cost and benefits of things. Is the $20 off of the heating tool really going to save you, or will you end up spending double or triple that purchasing items in an attempt to repair the damage that came from using low-quality products and tools on your hair? Most likely, the latter. Invest in products that work with great precision, so as to reduce the amount of work you have to do and the amount of damage you experience.

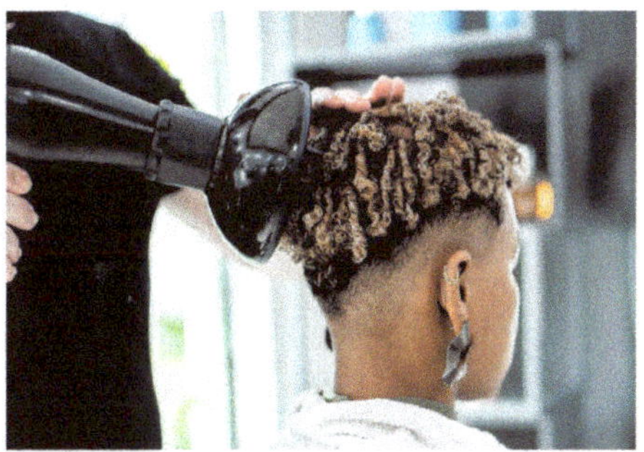

4. Blow-dryers are also a heating tool that should be used with caution. The proximity of the blow-dryer to the hair strand is crucial for protecting the hair. Please avoid pressing the end of the dryer directly against your hair. The direct heat as well as the physical contact on the heating elements of the dryer could not only lead to damage but possibly a fire. Allow for space between the heat and your precious locks.

Pro tip: Don't be afraid to use the cool-air setting! Your hair can dry with cool air, and it does not pose as great of a risk for your hair!

Chemicals

When considering the use of chemicals, one must proceed with caution. Similar to heat, chemical use often results in permanent outcomes. Altering the chemical makeup or composition of hair is not reversible, so prior to product use, proper research should be done in order to execute the style with minimal damage. There are two different kinds of common chemical treatments I am going to discuss with you—hair relaxers or texturizers and dyes.

Hair Relaxers / Texturizers

Looking beyond our preconceived notions in regard to these products, be it good or bad, there are some hard facts we must face. Hair relaxers are tools used by many people in order to attain straighter locks when heating tools alone do not suffice. Chemical relaxers work by breaking the disulfide bonds in the layer under the cuticle—the cortex. The release of disulfide bonds or the result of having less disulfide bonds in one's hair produces visibly straighter hair since the bonds are what is causing the extent of curliness of one's hair.

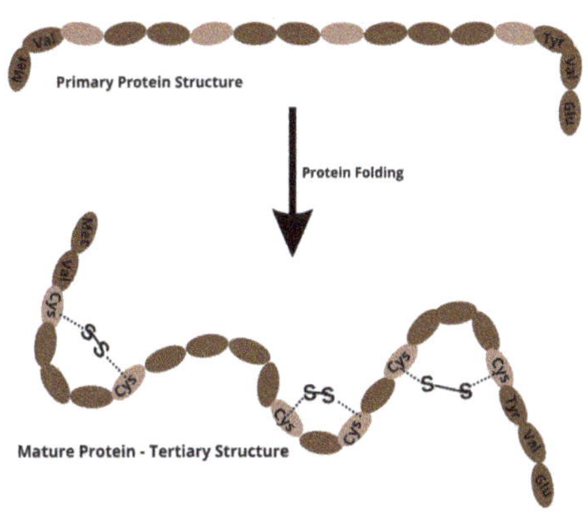

The curlier the hair, the stronger the chemical concoction must be in order to disrupt the cortex layer and alter hair texture. Using strong products can have more adverse reactions such as dryness, brittleness, breakage, and thinning. Since chemical relaxers have to penetrate through the cuticle, it is removing a much needed layer of protection from the hair, leaving it in a very vulnerable position.

In addition to its effects on the hair strands, chemical relaxers also penetrate the scalp and seep into the roots of the hair. Albeit, we have addressed the importance of caring for the hair from root to tip by ensuring products are applied thoroughly, this is an exception. In order to care for the hair from root to tip in regard to chemical relaxers, it is perti-nent that caution be exercised during its application. Three of the main ingredients in chemical relaxers, which are sodium hydroxide, ammonium thiogly-colate, and sodium thioglycolate, are all well-known skin irritants. These chemicals are known to cause a range of symptoms from stinging and skin redness to more severe conditions like chemical burns.

Dyes

Another chemical mixture that is commonly applied to the hair is dye. Hair-coloring agents work in a variety of ways and include different concoctions of chemicals. The hair-coloring process results from many chemical reactions between the pigments and molecules in the hair as well as ammonia and peroxide.

It is important to note that not all hair-coloring methods have the same effect on hair. From natural hair colorants to temporary hair color, lightening and lastly permanent hair color, there are a lot of options for those looking to switch up their hair color. While most of these hair-coloring methods involve opening up the hair shaft in order to reform new chemical bonds, natural hair colorants apply color directly to the hair shaft. Because they do not open the hair shaft, this can be more gentle on the strands and help prevent excessive drying. My favorite hair-coloring tool is henna. This mineral-rich product also seconds as hair dye. In conjunction with teas and coffees, a variety of colors can be achieved by using henna.

In contrast to natural colorants and some temporary color agents, permanent color can only be deposited into the hair once the cuticle layer has been opened. The chemical that opens the cuticle is ammonia, also the same ingredient used for hair lightening, found in bleach. The second chemical in use is peroxide, which is used as the developer in order to remove preexisting color. Peroxide is the scissors which cuts/breaks sulfur-containing chemical bonds, creating the distinctive hair dye odor.

Fix/Solution

When it comes to the use of any chemicals on the hair and body, it is pertinent that adequate research is done to find out exactly what products are contained and what the proper application method is. You are the expert on you, so get to know yourself and what works best for you. Also be aware that chemical alterations are going to be irreversible or permanent because they are altering the chemical makeup of the hair.

There are some methods or tips and tricks you can use as an attempt to protect your hair when engaging with chemicals.

1. First and foremost, invest time in reading the instructions. In today's world of instant this or instant that, it might slip your mind to read the three-page pamphlet inside the box but *DON'T*! The product manufacturers are the most well versed on the product, its ingredients, and the possible adverse reactions. Their guide has been written to help you not only achieve the perfect style or color you're going for but also to protect you along the way.

2. Begin with hair and a scalp that is healthy. If you are currently experiencing issues such as excessively dry scalp or dandruff, it is important that you begin by addressing the issues at hand prior to using any chemicals. Most chemicals have their own adverse reaction such as dryness and brittleness, so adding them to an unhealthy scalp will only exacerbate the issues you're currently dealing with.

3. Apply relaxers to "dirty hair" or at least hair that is not freshly washed. This point also echoes the first tip—*read the instructions* because mostly all of these products inform the user of the importance of applying the chemicals on hair that isn't clean. Hair naturally produces lots of healthy oils.

Chemicals like relaxers strip the hair of all of those oils in order to penetrate the cuticle, so having a layer of oils on the hair will prevent excessive stripping, providing the hair with a small layer of protection.

4. Avoid application on the scalp. I know, I know. This one you didn't want to hear. Albeit, the goal might also be to get slick edges, you might want to reconsider honey. Knowing that the three main ingredients are also notorious skin irritants should be enough of a deterrent, if it's not you might want to consider adding another protective layer to your hair prior to chemical application. Applying a protective base on the scalp, like petroleum jelly, can go a long way in preventing dryness and chemical burns.

5. Don't overuse them. Anything done in excess can ultimately be detrimental, so don't overdo it. From chemical relaxers to dyes and colorants, it is important to use these products in moderation. Allow time to pass before reapplying chemicals to the hair.

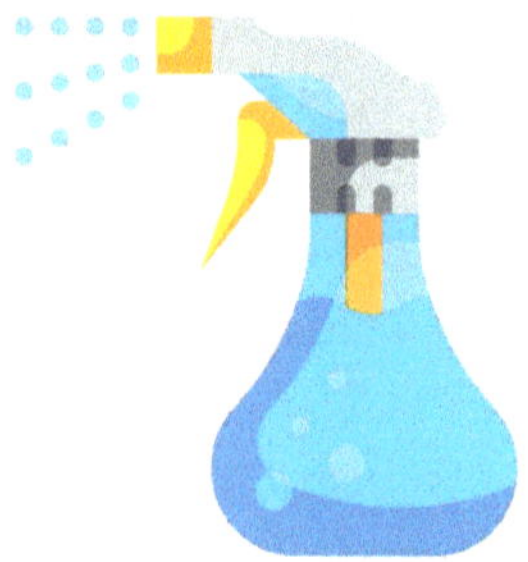

6. Moisture. Moisture. Moisture. Yet again moisture is the answer to our hair issues. Because chemicals strip the hair and open the cuticle, the hair becomes prone to drying without that layer of protection. To combat this, you must add and maintain high levels of moisture in the hair. Adding moisturizing products such as conditioners and sealing with oil will help reseal the cuticle and aid in moisture retention. Stay consistent with your moisturizing regimen when altering your hair in any way.

Chapter 6

Protective Styles

The topic of protective styles rides under "minimal breakage," but because this is such an extensive subject, it is deserving of its own chapter.

I'd like to begin this section with a *myth buster!*

Rumor: "Protective styles are styles that last for four to six weeks with little-to-no maintenance, often leaving the hair without water or fertilization (oils at the roots) for the sake of maintaining a style."

Busted: This is a myth! Styles like the one described above are simple styles that put the hair away, not necessarily "protective."

Protective styles are used for growth and maintaining hair health, keep the hair and ends away in order to prevent unnecessary breakage, and allow for proper root-to-tip moisturization of hair. Upon observation of all other areas of the human body, which are covered in hair for both males and females, it is evident that water is necessary for rapid hair growth. The whole body—legs, back, arms, chest, and even face—is covered in hair, which receives a daily (typically) dousing of water; logically, that sometimes pesky hair seems to experience never-ending hair growth. Illogically, how can one expect the hair on the head to grow in the absence of regular watering? Regardless of hairstyle—the hair should never be deprived of water!

As far as fertilizing, nutrients need to be given to the hair and scalp on a regular basis. Nutrients for the hair can come in the form of oil and grease among a variety of other products. They should be applied to both the scalp and hair in varying amounts and degrees of consistency. Without these products, the hair is deprived of additional nutrients outside of water.

Regardless of hairstyle—the hair should never be deprived of nutrients!

Not all protective styles are created the same. Different styles provide different levels of protection for the locks in question. In the sections below, we will unravel the truths about these styles and the best techniques to instill during the use of each.

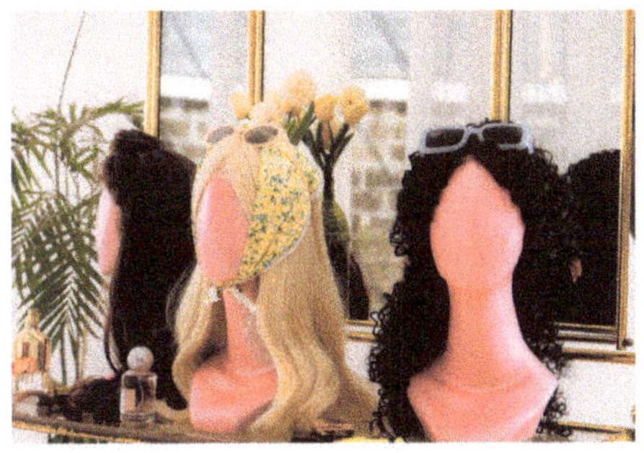

Wigs

Depending on the installation method, wigs can fall quite short of the mark of truly being "protective." The style of wig I would be most concerned about are "sew-in full lace wigs"—wigs made with caps that prevent direct access to the scalp. This is detrimental to hair health because like plant health, it is significantly dependent on the health of its roots. So limiting access to something like the life source (like an umbilical cord for a developing child) for the hair also limits overall hair health. Optimal moisture levels are difficult to achieve in this style since water is not applied directly to the hair or scalp. Watering also has to be kept at minimal levels because of the challenge to thoroughly dry all of the hair in order to prevent mold growth (in extreme cases). Likewise to the complications arising from limited access to the scalp for watering, fertilizing the roots shares in the added difficulty caused by the "temporarily permanent" (until the removal of the wig when sewn in) cap.

There are some tips and tricks you can put to use in order to rock your desired styles with confidence in its ability to protect your hair.

Here are some tips to try:

1. Opt for the Non-Sewn Version
    Glueless wigs are an excellent option. I love them because their easy removability allows for quick and constant access to the scalp and hair for regular maintenance. These wigs often come with an elastic band that is meant to replace glue or glue-like product use, adding an additional benefit to the hairline.
    When the elastic band of the glueless option is unavailable, a non-aggressive glued-on wig would be fine. "Nonaggressive" can, at times, refer to "weaker" products. In this case, I am referring to glues which aren't as strong and might require more frequent reapplication. I recommend choosing "stronghold" gels instead of more typical hair glues.

2. Short-Term Wear
    In regard to wigs, I define *short term* as two to three days (at most, four days) of wearing prior to removal. Choosing less aggressive glue-like products allows for easier

removal and more constant hair and scalp maintenance.

3. Don't Forget About Those Edges or That Kitchen!
    The hair located on the front and back hairline can be quite fragile. It is important to include them in what gets protected within a hairstyle.

Pro tip: Use something silk under the wig to protect the edges from the friction created by movement of the wig or wig cap during use.

Be sure to also be weary of the elastic band. It too produces friction during wig use, which can result in unwanted breakage of the back hairline/nape of neck hair.

Pro tip: Try adding silk to your elastic band for added protection with reduced pullage from friction.

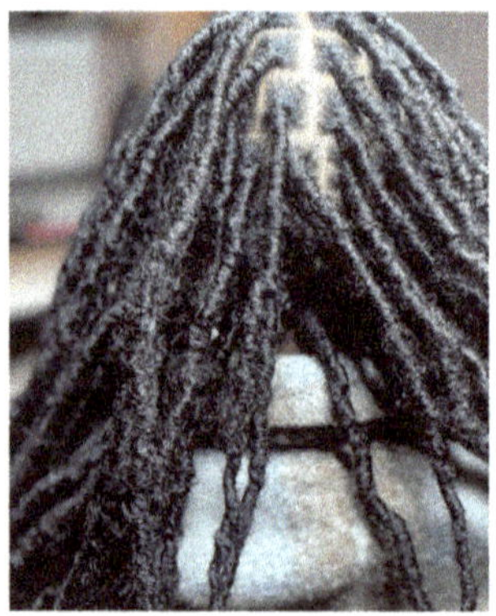

Braids with Extensions

Braids with extensions are a style adored by many naturals from youth and even onto early and late adulthood. With their resemblance to hair strands, they do offer great versatility in styling while also permitting a good level of hair care maintenance. There are numerous tactics which can be put to use in conjunction with styles that fit into this category in order to maintain good levels of hair health.

Here are a few tips to consider:

1. Cater to the Extensions Prior to Installation Anything that comes in packaging from an unknown warehouse should be cleaned prior to its placement on your being. Most hair extensions originate in faraway lands and pass through the hands of many before arriving

on one's doorstep. Both human and synthetic hair should be treated prior to its combining with one's natural hair. I recommend cleaning the hair for both physical and spiritual cleanliness. Your crown is the gateway to your entire being through the portal that is your mind. Be mindful of the things you adorn on your crown because that energy is transmitted throughout your body from your mind.

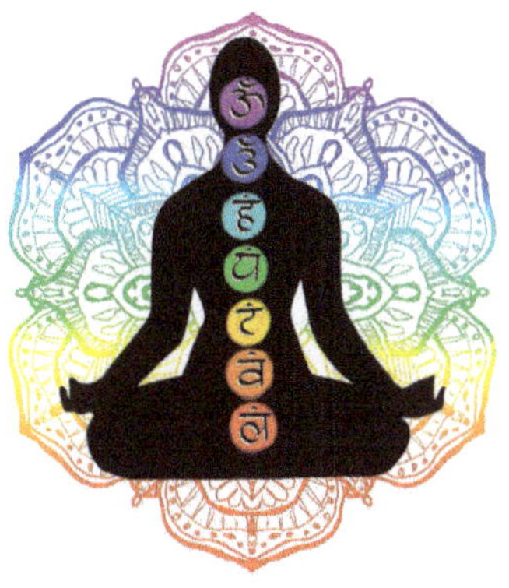

2. Do Not Get Attached to the Idea of the Style Maintaining That "Fresh Look"
    We all feel amazing with a fresh and crisp style, but it is important to not let the desire to maintain that newness overpower the desire to be a good plant mom/dad to the growing plant baby. Water will make the natural hair frizz up as the coils begin to

spring out of the braids, but have no fear! The compression from a scarf/durag can assist in taming the flying strands. There are also products like mousses and butters that also aid in slicking the style down. Regardless of that state of the style, slick or frizzy, you are beautiful.

Because of the importance of suitable hair and scalp fertilization, it can often be necessary to disrupt those perfectly crisp parts. Rubbing oil and/or grease on the scalp has the potential to remove strands from the braid, in turn creating frizz. The amount of frizz created can be reduced by way of the use of an oil applicator bottle in place of the fingers.

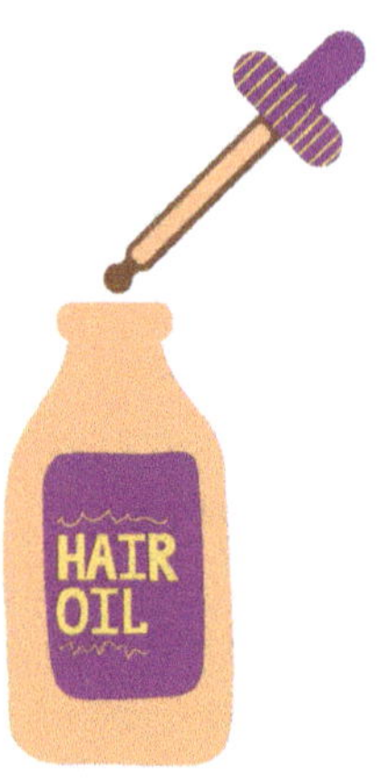

3. Wash Your Hair

Even during the use of protective styles, it is pertinent that the wash regime be maintained as well. The consistency in which hair needs to be washed is dependent on the unique elements of each individual's hair makeup. This is discussed in more detail in Chapter 2. If you are someone who washes your hair every two weeks, a box braid install should not change that. Maintaining the cleanliness of the hair helps reduce product and dead skin buildup, which is important in the removal of a style. Buildup bubbles form at the base of the braid, near the scalp, and can often lead to tangles and knots in the hair, so regular washes are necessary in order to keep these bubbles at bay.

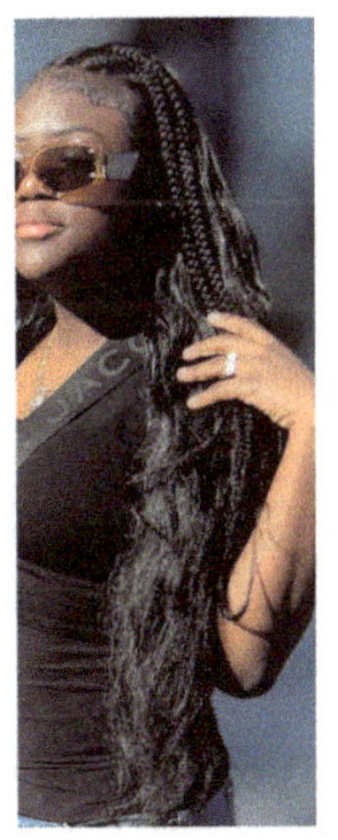

4. These Styles Are Supposed to Be *Temporary*

Do not attempt to stretch the wear of the style until it is on its last legs. Proper and regular hair care maintenance will result in styles that do not maintain freshness for two or more months. Do not be afraid to let the style go when it is beginning to grow out and create tension at the root of the hair strand. It is important to note that the longer the extensions, the shorter the wear should be. Longer braided or twisted extensions are heavier, especially when wet, resulting in a great amount of tension being applied to the hair and scalp. As the hair grows out and the natural hair becomes exposed at the root, breakage from the root becomes an even greater possibility with the hair in such a vulnerable position. I suggest a maximum of three weeks for time of wear of hip length and longer braids.

Twists, Locs, and Braids

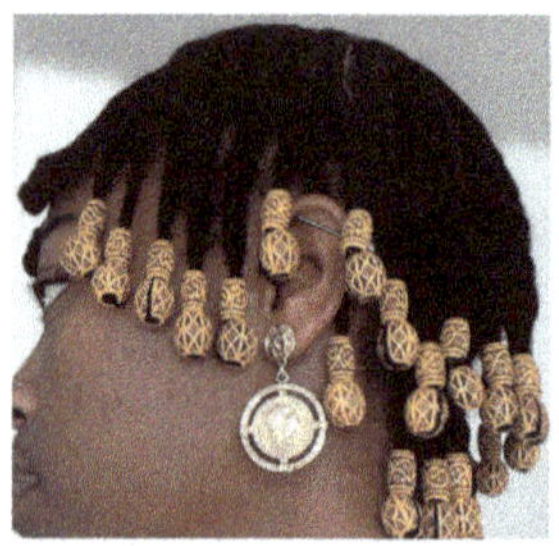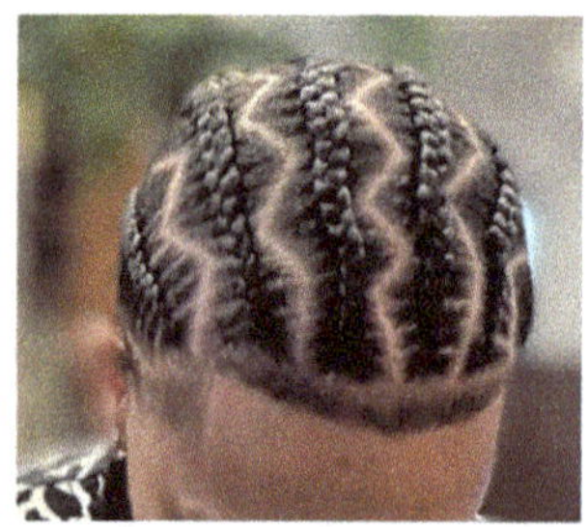

These are among my favorite and most highly recommended protective styles done without the use of extensions. The use of extensions for these styles is fine, as long as the "tips to consider" are used. Twists like two-strand twists, finger coils, and locs provide great versatility in styling while maintaining hair health and allowing for regular hair maintenance, similarly to braids like cornrows and flat twist which also provide excellent hair maintenance abilities and protection of the hair strand. Do not shy away from protective styles using your natural hair!

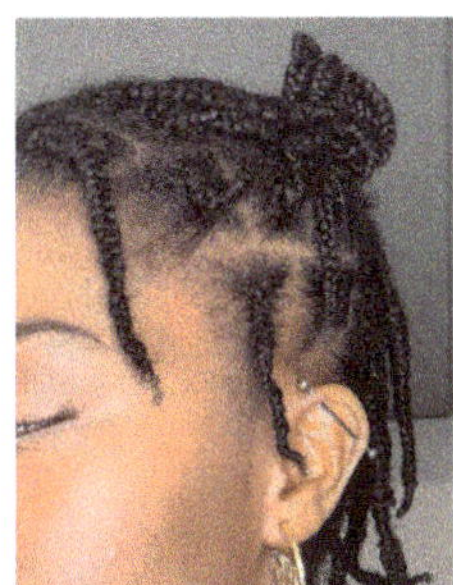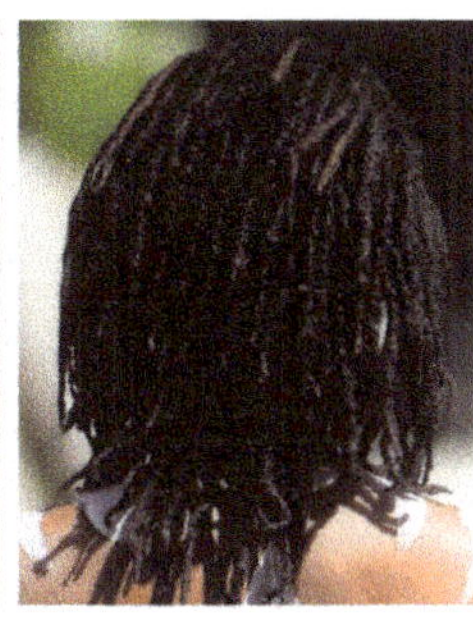

Chapter 7

Diet

The saying "you are what you eat" should be a proverb in every home. A major pathway for nutrients to enter the body is through the mouth. You choose if you want to ingest healing, edible substances, or ones with more detrimental effects on the body. Diet impacts all areas of health within the being, not excluding hair.

Protein is one of the most talked about macromolecules in today's society, rightfully so because of its vital role in almost every life-giving chemical reaction as well as its overall importance in the body's daily functions. The topic in question is not if protein is necessary or not. It is how much of it is required to maintain the subject in question (muscle mass, hair strength, or nail length). The answer to that inquiry isn't very simple because it is dependent on and influenced by a number of factors including but not limited to size, age, gender, degree of health, and desired outcome.

As someone who has been consuming a plant-based diet for the past five years, the questions "how do you get enough protein" and "where do you get protein from" have been posed to me so many times that one might think I'm running a nutrition course or something. This kind of query has always been interesting to me because for those ingesting "regular diets," ones including animal products, no one seems to be as concerned about their ability to maintain adequate levels of ingested proteins.

I'm here to say that protein is important for everyone, regardless of dietary restrictions, but also to say that protein is found in almost every food item. As surprising as this may be for some, there are a plethora of protein-rich fruits, vegetables, and starches. For both men and women, the average amount of protein required is 46–56 grams a day or the equivalent of 200–700 calories a day based on a 2,000-calorie diet. A range of 200–700 is very wide, so it is important to consider the many other factors that influence dietary protein requirement.

Did you know?: hair and nails grow at the same rate!

If your nails appear to be growing at a much faster rate than your hair, the rate of breakage might be equivalent to rate of growth (I recommend reviewing chapter 5, "Minimal Breakage"). It is also possible to experience periods in which the rate of growth is quicker for the hair than nails; in this case, you might be lacking in the amount and kind/quality of dietary proteins as well as other essential nutrients.

The healthiest sources of protein generally originate from plants. The right type of meat sources are also capable of providing quality nutrients when eaten in moderation. There are a number of protein sources you can choose from: soy, nuts, seeds, beans and lentils, skinless white-meat chicken or turkey, egg whites, whey protein, or fish. Protein-rich meals can look like the following:

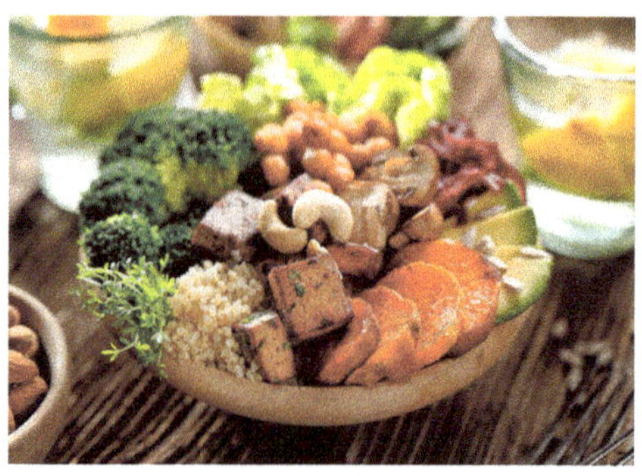

1. Banana, Greek yogurt, and egg = 19 grams of protein

2. 3-ounce chicken breast, half cup of rice, and half cup of veggies = 25 grams of protein

For those who aren't able to fulfill these dietary requirements with food, supplements could be of great use. Quality protein supplements should have no more than 200 calories, 2 grams of saturated fat, 5 grams of sugar, and no trans-fat or partially hydrogenated oils.

If you need further assistance with your diet, you should consider requesting the assistance of a nutritionist.

Conclusion

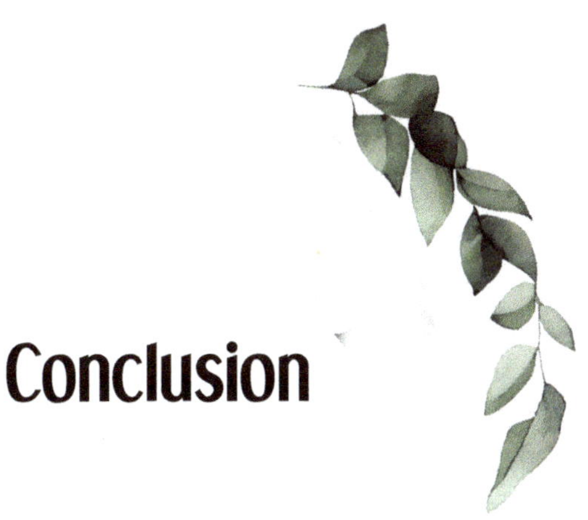

Thank you for joining me on this journey. Hair is beautiful and speaks volumes in the representation of who we are. Take the time to personally get to know your hair and all the magnificent kinks that make him or her who they are. Take your time and remember that the goal is growth: growth of hair health, growth of perspective, and growth of well-being.

Because every hair journey is individual to the head it is attached to, the products and methods that work best for me and my hair might not work well for your hair. Use the many resources available to you to compile as much information as you can in order to make the most educated assumptions and decisions about your hair. If you are experiencing medical complications or issues of the scalp, be sure to discuss these concerns with a medical provider.

I pray that this can aid in creating a greater amount of ease in the natural hair journey of all those who come across this.

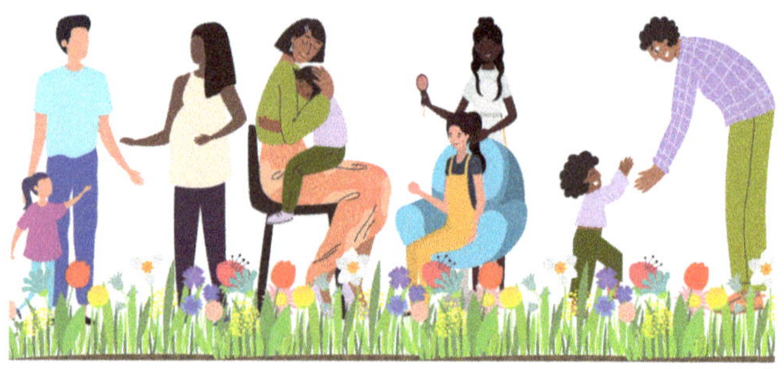

P.S.

To all mothers, fathers, guardians, and beauticians, this is for you.

Please, please, please be mindful of the words you use in regard to the locks arising from the heads of your precious little ones. Before they can form their own opinions of themselves and the world around them, they often adopt yours.

Refrain from saying things like "Oh my gosh, I hate doing his/her hair" or "Your hair is too thick" or anything else that insinuates the difficulty of managing hair like theirs or, worse yet, anything that might make them think that you do not like their hair. Statements like these affect the young minds of children more than we realize. Those ideas run through their minds and soon become things they unconsciously say to themselves.

In order to instill more love in the hearts and minds of children, it is important to consider your rhetoric and tone in interactions with them. Speak loving phrases as you embark on styling their hair:

- Your hair is beautiful.
- I am blessed with hands that are able to handle your hair.
- Doing your hair does not have to be painful.
- I have enough time to complete the style you desire.
- You having thick hair means more hair to love.
- I love watching thoughts turn to things as we create art in your hair.
- With adequate time and proper information, I have the tools necessary to do your hair.
- I will be patient with your hair.
- Your hair is manageable.
- I am grateful to spend this time with you.

Helping children realize their beauty in youth allows for strong-minded and confident adults to blossom. As their guardians, you are their first teachers. Please gift them with affirmations so those seeds will take root as self-love in the future.

Thank you for taking the time to learn about caring for their hair. I know they are in great hands.

I hope this helps.

With love,
Thembekile Dube

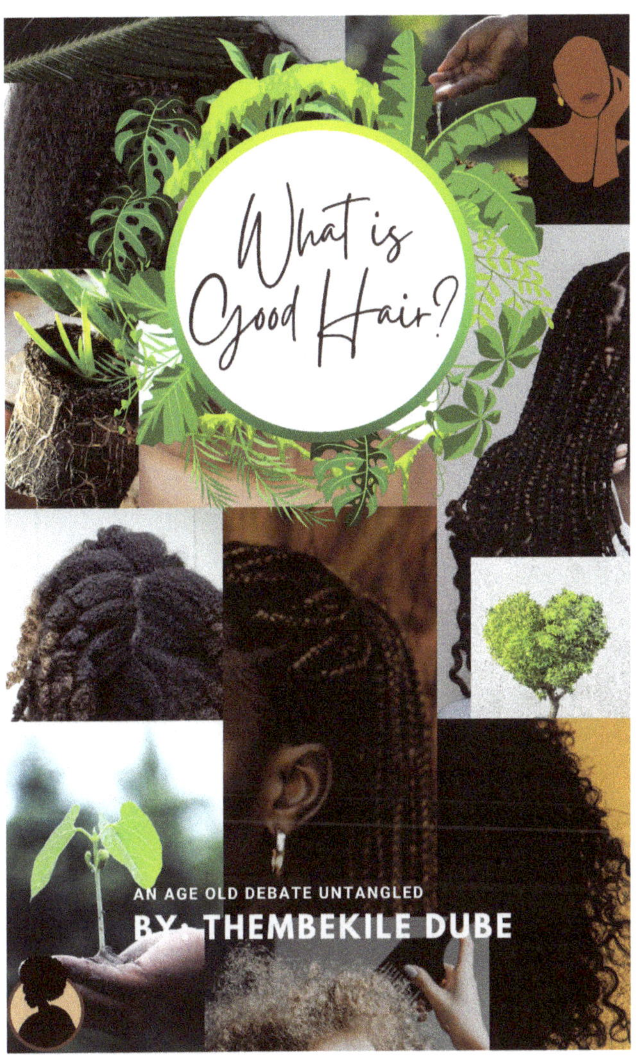
What is
Good Hair?
AN AGE OLD DEBATE UNTANGLED
BY THEMBEKILE DUBE

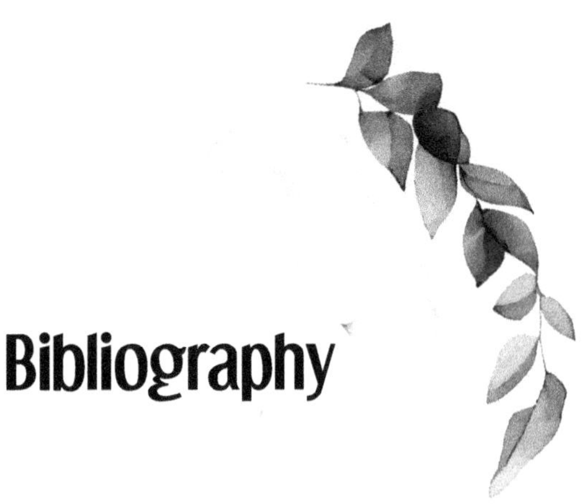

Bibliography

Dorfner, Micah. "Are You Getting Too Much Protein?—Mayo Clinic News Network." Mayo Clinic, Mayo Foundation for Medical Education and Research. November 7, 2018. https://newsnetwork.mayoclinic.org/discussion/are-you-getting-too-much-protein.

Dyson. "How Does Heat Damage Hair?" https://www.dyson.com/knowledge/hair-care/how-does-heat-damage-hair.

Glow, Hello. "5 Ways to Use Eggs for Healthier Hair." Pete and Gerry's Organic Eggs. June 6, 2019. https://www.peteandgerrys.com/blog/eggs-for-healthier-hair.

Gould, Hallie. "Avocado for Hair: Benefits and How to Use It." Byrdie. March 1, 2022. https://www.byrdie.com/avocados-for-hair.

Head and Shoulders. "Relaxers—How Do They Work?" https://headandshoulders.com/en-us/healthy-hair-and-scalp/hair-care/relaxers-how-do-they-work.

Helmenstine, Anne Marie, PhD. "The Science of Hair Coloring." ThoughtCo. August

27, 2020. https://www.thoughtco.com/salon-hair-color-chemistry-602183.

Medical News Today. "Avocado Oil for Hair: Benefits and How to Use It." MediLexicon International. https://www.medicalnewstoday.com/articles/321606#benefits.

———. "Mayonnaise Hair Mask: Benefits, How to Use, and More." MediLexicon International. https://www.medicalnewstoday.com/articles/mayonnaise-hair-mask#how-to-use-a-mayonnaise-mask.

Watson, Kathryn. "Banana Hair Mask Benefits, plus Recipes for Dry Hair and Dandruff." Healthline, Healthline Media. July 15, 2019. https://www.healthline.com/health/banana-hair-mask#recipes.

WebMD. "Essential Oils for Hair Care." https://www.webmd.com/beauty/natural-oils.

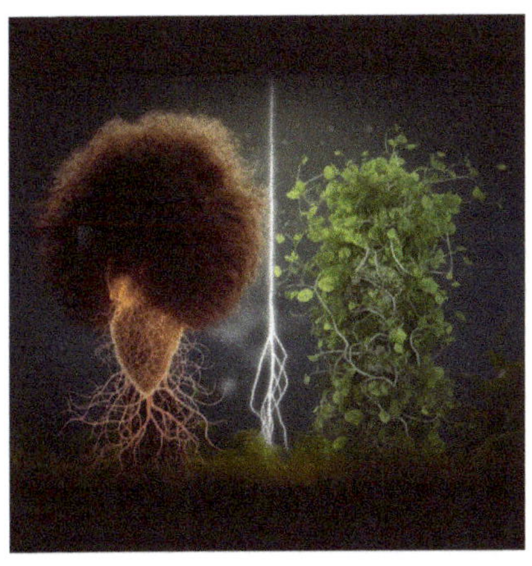

Hair

noun **threadlike growth of animate being**
synonym **plant, mane**

Similarities between hair and plants:
> ~ Strong yet vulnerable
> ~ (Almost) always growing
> ~ Reactive to elements in the environment
> ~ Root system functions as "heart" by pump-
> ing water and nutrients to the entire plant/
> head of hair

Treat your hair as you would a plant. Give it plenty of water and nutrients on a regular basis. Always be gentle when tending to those strands. Being kind also wouldn't hurt; try out the positive affirmations on page xiii.

I hope this helps

About the Author

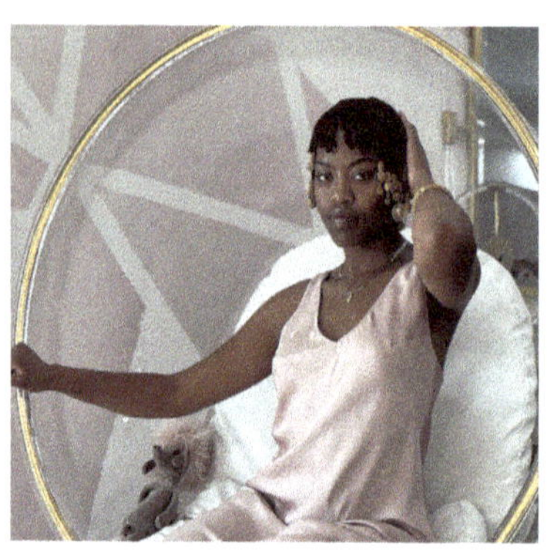

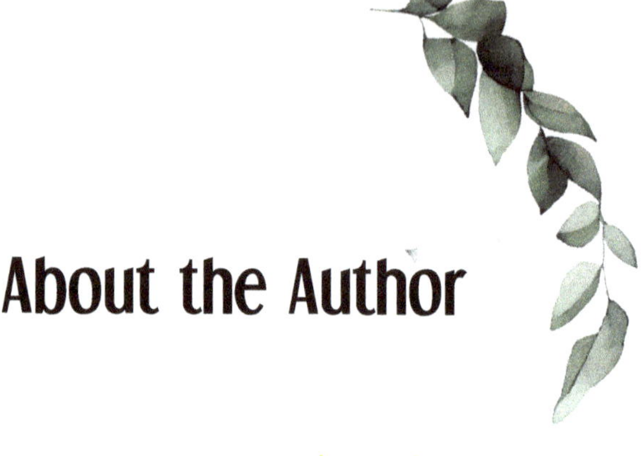

Thembekile Dube in Ndebele language means "trustworthy." Not only is that the meaning of her name, but that is the true content of her character. In her first nonfiction work, *What is Good Hair?*, she illuminates the reality of what taking care of hair like her own should entail.

A woman of many trades, she often finds it difficult to summarize her essence in concise literary text. With backgrounds in childcare, hair care, creative design and direction, writing, love, and biological sciences, she's what some (one being herself) might call "everything and a bag of chips." She lives by the philosophy that "life is easy," and in this book, she teaches readers how to make at least one aspect of their lives easier, that is, hair care. You can find out more about Thembekile and love at trustinlove.net.